C.F. NERO

Aftermath 2020

America Shaken

To my son, Breland

As you do graciously, daily you show me that I can overcome any fear, learn, and press on.

Contents

Preface

When life gives us lemons, we do not always feel like making lemonade. As humans, we can experience doubt, confusion, and even vexation before making certain decisions. We ponder over which decisions lead to the best possible outcomes. Our personal health is one of the most important aspects of our lives. When it comes to being an effective individual for our families, friends, colleagues, and communities, we must have wellness to do so. When an airborne illness threatens our life and livelihood, choices seem limited, and if given, often difficult to make.

The purpose for this book is to briefly examine key moments of the COVID pandemic that forced intense, life-altering decisions. It discusses how American citizens navigated murky waters, suffering and persevering amid setbacks and devastation. The reader will receive highlights and perspectives on how division over coerced health choices almost tore families, communities, and society at large, in pieces. At the core, this book delves into the impact of mandated personal health decisions on the masses. It addresses how media messaging can work to bring harmony or conspire to create unproductive feuding. The question to ask is, "Were the measures solely instituted for the safety of the public or was this practice (a test run) for another agenda?". Motives must be unveiled for the American people to trust the plans implemented in the name of their health and well-being. It has been proven that mandates and coerced compliance accompany consequences with lasting impact.

1

The Occurrence

Reflections from December of 2019 encompassed the sound of Christmas carols, businesses with joyful shoppers, and the wonderful smell of freshly prepared meals. There were lists made, gifts purchased to wrap, and many travel plans underway. It was presumed to be a typical holiday that families were elated to enjoy. These were among the memories that filled American hearts and minds. Reminiscing the season, appreciation of what was a simple and carefree time, warms the soul. Unknown to many, the 2019 holiday season would be one to truly cherish, as America and the world was headed toward the edge of a precipice.

A horrid illness swept the country, announced to be Coronavirus disease (COVID-19). COVID-19 is an infectious disease caused by the SARS-CoV-2 virus. COVID-19, according to Johns Hopkins Medicine, emerged in December of 2019 causing mild symptoms for some, and more moderate to severe symptoms for others. Symptoms included cough, fever, shortness of breath, muscle and body aches, loss of taste and smell, fatigue, congestion, and more. There were also individuals who were unknowing asymptomatic carriers of the virus.

Numerous sources, including the Centers for Disease Control and Prevention (CDC), believed that Wuhan, China was the possible origin of this novel coronavirus infection. This belief was accounted to the World Health Organization (WHO) Country Office in China informing of various cases of pneumonia with symptoms of fever and shortness of breath. At the time, these initial cases in Wuhan were connected back to their Huanon Seafood Wholesale Market. The city of Wuhan, with a population of 11 million people, was placed on lockdown January 23, 2020. The country of China informed of its' first COVID-19 death in January of 2020. The United States also confirmed its' first COVID-19 patient the same month. The World Health Organization (WHO) declared a global health emergency on January 30, 2020. The first COVID-19 death in the United States was reported in February of 2020.

On March 11, 2020, the World Health Organization (WHO) declared COVID-19 to be a pandemic. Reportedly, across numerous countries, there were more than 115,000 cases, and almost 5,000 deaths. On March 12, 2020, the first COVID-19 restrictions were issued in America. This resulted from an outbreak around the area of New Rochelle, New York. The orders to quarantine and shelter-in-place were given to anyone exposed, or possibly exposed, to an infected individual for an initial 14-day timeframe. Former President Trump declared a national emergency on March 13, 2020. Flights were restricted to and from certain areas where the disease was detected. Cruises were also docked and cancelled from numerous passenger infections. As more American states began to experience an influx of ill citizens, more government officials begin implementing protective measures in their cities and states. This included full lockdowns for everyone except emergency and essential workers. Schools and non-essential businesses across the nation were closed as well. Some states were stricter than others, with longer lengths of COVID-19 restrictions. President Trump charged most decisions regarding the public's health to be in the hands of each state's governor, believing they more effectively knew their residents and data regarding infection and hospital rates.

Many efforts were instituted in attempt to lower hospital admissions. There were simply not enough beds or staff to service the ill patients needing dire treatment. Ventilators and continuous care were necessary. Hospital supply shortages were rampant. There were significant country-wide hospitalizations and deaths from the respiratory disease. It wreaked havoc on those with comorbidities and senior citizens. Physicians and nurses were regularly interviewed on news media outlets urging citizens to only go necessary places, follow all CDC guidelines, and governmental mandates in effort to slow the spread of the virus. According to CDC data charts, from the years 2020 to 2023, the largest amount of American people hospitalized with COVID-19 were in the age groups of 18 to 49 and 65 years and older. Seniors passed away at very alarming numbers. In the year 2020, over 66 percent of COVID-19 deaths were among those aged 65 years and older. By late September of 2020, the United States death toll from COVID-19 surpassed 200,000 people. On May 12, 2022, the CDC reported the recorded death toll from COVID in America to be at a disturbing 1 million people.

2

Health Decisions

COVID-19 caused a widespread haze. Aside from quarantining, American citizens were perplexed as to what to do, and how to respond, if and when they did contract the illness. Questions and concerns regarding contraction, immunity, treatments, and overall wellness, were unanswered. The public needed to know if COVID-19 was only contracted by touch of surfaces, or was it also transmitted in the air. Discussions surged around public mask and glove usage. Various government officials and scientists would make interview appearances on news media platforms stating that masks were not needed or required in public places. Only healthcare workers were said to need them. By April of 2020, masks became recommended for all who were over the age of 2 years old in public settings. The CDC confirmed in July of 2020 that the masks would likely contribute to preventing transmission of the virus. This concurred with the belief that the virus was airborne the entire time. Unsettling as the confirmation was, many Americans were relieved that they could do something to prevent contraction and spread. Opponents were suspicious of mask wearing effectivity. The N95 surgical masks were the most protectant masks to wear. These particular masks sold out due to high demand from healthcare industry workers. Cloth masks or masks without filters, would not sufficiently protect against the contagious viral particles. It was also recommended to wear more than one mask at a time. In January of 2021, President Biden signed numerous executive orders, one of which required facial masking for all American travel to include airports, ships, airplanes, and public transportation.

The standard listed by the CDC to prevent coronavirus transmission became six foot social or physical distancing when in essential places such as grocery stores or work sites. This clashed with the World Health Organization (WHO) who required three feet. Pfizer sources stated that other scientists recommended further distancing. They cited that respiratory droplets could travel as far as 23 to 27 feet.

At onset, simple, general advice was given to manage COVID-19 symptoms upon contraction. The quandary was that there was no provided medical advice on medications for this illness. Information was relayed to increase sunlight, stay hydrated, and to take the supplements Vitamin D and Zinc. Some medical experts recommended cold and influenza over the counter cough syrup, along with pain and fever reducers. For excessive coughing, cough syrup was prescribed. It was not recommended to initially use antivirals such as Remdesivir. In September of 2020, the Journal of the American Medical Association and the World Health Organization (WHO) began recommending the use of steroids for the treatment of severe COVID-19 disease. Multiple studies found that steroids such as dexamethasone, hydrocortisone, and methylprednisolone reduced mortality in these severe cases of infection by up to 36 percent.

The first human trials for a vaccine were underwent in Seattle, Washington by Moderna Therapeutics in March of 2020. Operation Warp Speed was introduced under the Trump Administration on April 30, 2020. Its effort was to produce a vaccine against the virus swiftly, to curtail further excessive hospitalizations and limit deaths. By August 17, 2020, the CDC cited that COVID-19 became the third leading cause of

American deaths. The death toll exceeded 1,000 people per day. Obesity also became a high-risk issue for mortality from the virus across all racial, socioeconomic, or ethnic backgrounds. On December 11, 2020, Pfizer-BioNTech's vaccine was U.S. Food and Drug Administration (FDA) approved for emergency use in individuals 16 years and older to prevent the spread of COVID-19. Deliveries began within days. On December 18, 2020, the FDA issued authorization to Moderna for persons aged 18 years and older. Months later, on February 27, 2021, the third emergency authorization was given for the Johnson & Johnson COVID-19 vaccine in those aged 18 years and older.

Concerns emerged around the pharmaceutical industry acting so abruptly to produce and release vaccines for this novel virus. There was also speculation of the overall safety of these particular vaccines. Critics believed there to be a profit motive at work. Per a July of 2022 Kaiser Health News report, Pfizer's 2021 revenue amassed $81.3 billion, of which $7.8 billion being United States revenue. The creation and release of vaccines came too soon for skeptics, and for others, it was believed a godsend. Certain Americans were "in the middle" on the issue, as they were vaccine receivers against influenza, mumps, rubella, and other illnesses, however, indecisive on this one. Many people were simply desperate for a hopeful return to "normalcy".

An interesting observation was that some Christians voiced belief of the vaccine possibly being the actual mark of the beast (as mentioned in the Bible's book of Revelation 13). Others, as I, believed that this particular inoculation presented as one of many upcoming "precursors" that would desensitize the mind (through fear, ridicule, and intimidation), coerce, and ready the masses for other grave things to come (by force) in the foreseeable future. In that regard, the opinion was, and for some still is, that this vaccine was an initial checkmate maneuver on the pathway towards citizens accepting the New World Order's coming mandates.

Commonplace discussions in households were whether senior aged relatives were healthy enough for this vaccine, and if the youth should be inoculated as well. There were reports of small percentages of citizens having adverse reactions to the Johnson & Johnson, Moderna, and Pfizer vaccines. These symptoms included tiredness, headache, muscle aches, swelling, rashes, fever, chills, and more. The CDC noted that these adverse occurrences were rare. According to initial information, citizens who received full vaccination, would not contract the virus. It was also broadcasted that even though an individual may have had the virus, they needed to receive the vaccines too, as there was no immunity built against future infection. Any position or vocalized thoughts on herd immunity, were publicly discredited. The inceptive finding was that there was at least six months to a year of immunity after inoculation. Over time, as breakthrough infections were studied, an article from Johns Hopkins Medicine presented that out of 4 million plus fully vaccinated people, 1 in 100 people had a breakthrough COVID-19 infection between January 17, 2021 to August 21, 2021. A May of 2022 report from OSF Healthcare, posited that those who were fully vaccinated had a lower viral load if they did become infected.

On September 22, 2021, the FDA gave emergency authorization for a single Pfizer-BioNTech booster dose to be administered six months after the original doses of the vaccine for those aged 65 years and older, individuals aged 18 to 64 years who are at high risk of severe COVID-19, and those aged 18 to 64 years old who have frequent institutional or occupational travel, giving higher exposure to the disease. The World Health Organization (WHO) defined "Long COVID" as the continual or development of new symptoms three months after the initial SARS-CoV-2 infection. These symptoms must last at least two months following infection with no other explanation. A June 7, 2023 article from Yale Medicine informed that they have a Long COVID program aimed towards treating patients with lingering symptoms to include fatigue, brain fog, and shortness of breath. Research remains unclear on the exact percentage of American citizens suffering with this condition. It is also a condition that affects anyone, regardless of age, race, ethnicity, or socioeconomic background. In May of 2023, a news release from the National Institute of Health (NIH) revealed that a dozen people with persistent neurological symptoms after SARS-CoV-2 infections were studied and found to have differences in their autonomic dysfunction and immune cell profiles. The comprehensive testing of this group of people allowed for future testing to determine accurate diagnoses and possible treatments.

Amid vaccine productions, face masking, city curfews, social distancing measures and other mandates, variants of COVID-19 raised more questions as to the efficacy of these particular inoculations. The virus continued to evolve and transfer among the vaccinated and unvaccinated alike. A prevalent issue was that not everyone who contracted the virus displayed symptoms. One would have inferred that the vaccines may have needed updating to match the new variants, for effectiveness' sake.

In December of 2019, the known COVID-19 strain in circulation was called the L Strain. From this initial traced infection, the virus continued to change by replicating itself and creating a myriad of mutations. These mutations became variants of the original COVID-19 virus. Research shows that towards the end of 2020, the Alpha (B.1.1.7) variant was the cause of infection surges around the world. It was more deadly than the original L strain of COVID-19. Initially, the three major vaccines, Pfizer, Moderna, and Johnson & Johnson were effective against it.

The Beta (B.1.351) variant was identified in South Africa and spread quickly throughout Europe. Although it was 50 percent more transmissible, the vaccines still showed efficacy against this variant. The Gamma (P.1) variant had little effect on the American population. By July of 2020, a new variant appeared in southern California called Epsilon (B.1.427 and B.1.429). The reason for the World Health Organization's (WHO) unease was that the mutations in the spike protein enabled it

8

to maneuver around the antibodies people had from previous COVID infections and from the vaccines. As a result, the virus was transmitted easier. Kappa (B.1.617.1), Lambda (C.37), Eta (B.1.525), and Mu (B.1621, B.1.621.1) variants were more dominant outside of the United States. These were highly contagious and unresponsive to the vaccines. In February of 2021, Iota (B.1.526) and Zeta (P.2) variants were identified. In America, Iota was noticed in New York City and was perturbing due to citizens presenting heightened levels of symptoms from infection, along with a higher COVID mortality rate than the previous variants.

The Delta (B.1.617.2) variant brought further devastation in the spring of 2021. It spread across hundreds of countries causing startling numbers of hospitalizations and deaths. This variant affected the fully vaccinated and those who had already contracted and recovered from previous COVID infection. Reports showed over 70 percent of infections were breakthrough infections. Omicron (BA.1) was identified in the fall of 2021 and became more dominant than the Delta variant. It also composed several different subvariants throughout 2022. Omicron was difficult to detect because it mainly situated in the upper respiratory tract instead of moving into the lungs. The push from vaccine makers was to receive another booster shot as they begin to research and update versions of their vaccines against this variant. The FDA authorized Pfizer and Moderna's bivalent booster shots in September of 2022. According to information listed with the U.S. Department of Health and Human Services (DHHS), as of December 9, 2022 the CDC expanded COVID-19 vaccines to include children aged 6 months to 5 years old.

3

Social Ramifications

While Americans managed a major health crisis (with the information provided), social undertones brewed. The family, employment, and educational frameworks were challenged, and often strained. In its' initial phases, there were some couples who enjoyed the time to work from home. Many were non-essential workers who had the option. Couples with children were able to work online and the children could be supervised more attentively. Non-essential working families in 2020 were able to learn each other again, breaking from the hustle and bustle of commuting. Family activities and mealtimes were prioritized. Research presented from Bowling Green State University showed that the expectancy of divorces in 2020 was over 714,000 in the United States; however, only about 630,500 divorced, resulting in a 12 percent reduction.

According to a January 21, 2022 report from CNBC network, the disagreements over COVID restrictions were a wedge driver in families. A common issue of conflict was between parents who had varying outlooks on COVID and how it affected their children. One parent would be pro-COVID vaccination, and the other would be skeptical of it. Another voiced concern was if children should eventually be homeschooled or go back to attending regular school and childcare settings. Further accounts revealed that reluctant parents who did go through with allowing their children to be COVID vaccinated, regretted it later. Daunting decisions were faced, wondering if it was safe or a threatening exposure for adult children to visit with their senior aged parents. Another worry was if grandchildren (possibly carriers) should visit with their senior aged grandparents from March of 2020 through early 2022. Family parties and reunions were postponed, or cancelled, due to limitations or prohibitions of gathering in large numbers.

Americans experienced anxiety and overall fear from decisions passed down through officials. The grief of unexpected deaths took a toll on many households where relatives and friends were separated from one another during the pandemic. Countless stories of increased depression, anxiety, drug, alcohol abuse, and even self-deletion were reported during lockdowns. Women were stated to have the highest percentage of anxiety and depression. A February of 2023 article from Nationwide Children's Hospital-Center for Suicide Prevention and Research, informed that suicide was the second leading cause of death for individuals aged 5 to 24 years old in the United States. Suicide, in comparison to drug overdoses and homicides, declined to under 46,000 people, per the CDC. Many untreated mental health sufferers reverted to drug usage as a coping mechanism. Fentanyl overdoses largely increased. Allegedly over 106,000 people died as a result of drug overdose in 2021. On March 20, 2023, information from the Kaiser Family Foundation presented that almost three years after the onset of the pandemic, around 90 percent of American adults believed the country was still facing a mental health crisis.

Crime manifested in phases during the pandemic period. At onset of the 2020 lockdown, crime decreased across populated cities as a result of limited mobility. As time passed, the stay-at-home orders and business closures resulted in a reduction of home burglaries but increases in commercial break-ins and car thefts. Several articles relayed that the blame for criminal activity should be placed on the lockdowns themselves and not the virus. According to a January of 2023 report from CBS News, motor vehicle thefts across thirty major cities increased almost 60 percent from the years 2019 to 2022. This was a noticeable spike, as they were previously declining since the 1990s. Washington, DC experienced a heavy influx of carjackings and assaults. It was as if there was a repressed frustration and rage, unleashing itself at any given time or place. In the years 2020 and 2021, the location with the highest murder and negligent manslaughter was Memphis, Tennessee. By June 30, 2022, New Orleans, Louisiana had 145 murders alone. There were hundreds of brutal stabbings and shootings in cities like New York City, Chicago, Los Angeles, and other populated areas. Riding subways or public buses was found less safe than pre-pandemic. Gun violence skyrocketed. Some sources postulated that this was due to a sense of hopelessness and feared "loss of control" behind events affiliated with the pandemic.

With all of the pressing social dilemmas, a boiling issue was affecting the country daily. Since 2021, illegal immigration increased exponentially. In March of 2022, the U. S. Department of Homeland Security (DHS) advised that the average daily number of migrant crossings was at about 7,000 people. With such high volumes of undocumented people entering the United States at once, one viable apprehension from critics was that the migrants were not subjected to the same COVID coercions and requirements that American citizens endured. Certain news outlets were quiet concerning migrants' need to wear masks, quarantine, or receive vaccinations before entering or traveling throughout the United States.

The U. S. Department of Homeland Security's Customs and Border Protection is responsible for "securing" the American border from all potential threats. How could they do this while understaffed and without having the vital resources needed? Critics noted that the Biden Administration, to include Vice President Harris (the U. S. Border Czar), did not appear to view the Mexico- United States border being overrun as a violation of the proper procedure for entry, nor as a safety threat to American citizens. Supporters of these undocumented border crossers referred to the migrants as "asylum seekers". The state of Texas began, and continues to arrange, methods of transport for these incoming migrants out of their state. The governor of Texas and other officials expressed that they can no longer afford to solely carry the financial load of the numerous needs of illegal crossers. Many citizens wondered where the funds were coming from to clothe, feed, house, transport, and train these migrants.

Complaints swarmed as American veterans were going without, while undocumented migrants received an abundance of resources. Millions of tax dollars were allocated toward these individuals who had not yet contributed into the system they were pulling from. The cities of Chicago and New York City were regarded as major "sanctuary cities". Each city's mayor (already unsuccessfully handling their own city's crime escalation and resource limitation), went out of their way to accommodate migrants, defying the requests of their city's residents concerning their own homelessness/housing crisis and safety issues. The migrants were housed in hotels, shelters, closed schools, and other buildings. It did not take long before residents of these sanctuary cities cited the horrors of enhanced crime. They claimed to see children and teenagers being unaccompanied all hours of the night drinking, using drugs, having sex, and committing theft. Americans also began to notice that the most vocal advocates of the mass arrival of migrants, did not live near, or work around these "asylum seekers". These advocates put on "rose colored glasses", criticizing skeptics as inhumane and heartless if they dare mentioned anything about the migrants needing to go through the process that other legal immigrants have to complete (for the sake of equality and fairness). It was obvious that the migrants were not simply "passing through" the country for work opportunities. It was clear that they came to stay, thus the need to do it the lawful way. Those who were and are in proximity with the migrants, exposed the unrestrained lifestyle issues and lawlessness some brought with them across the border.

By 2023, the facade was over. Various sanctuary city residents were angry and tired of feeling ousted and fearful in their own neighborhoods. Although initially praised by various media platforms for risking it all to come to the United States, opponents knew the migrants would be pushed into low and middle income residential areas (without the consent of those residents). The city leaders refused to acknowledge the already high crime level as a deterrent for why migrants should not come in mass to those areas. The scales fell from Americans eyes as they witnessed when migrants were transferred from overwhelmed southern states to the affluent and resource rich areas of Washington, DC and Massachusetts. The migrants were "quickly" rerouted away. It was much easier to "vocalize" illegal immigration support on social platforms and across news outlets, for "social brownie points". When it came down to "actions", the resources of the wealthy acted swiftly to remove the migrants they beckoned to come. It was as if the opulent activists' silent stance was, "Alright now, you can come to America, but don't move near me and mine."

A final unsettling societal issue was pandemic school closures. Prolonged school closures were an area of newness for school aged children, forcing them to navigate online learning. While some children benefited, whether this be accounted to physical disability or general preference for virtual learning, other children were beset educationally and socially during the pandemic's school closures. Some children were fortunate to have what all children should, attentive parents. These parents actively monitored and assisted with their child's educational needs, ensuring that the child grasped each subjects' concepts, and completed all assignments. Unfortunately, there were students who did not have parental involvement in their education. These students required a more "hands on" approach and the accountability factor a structured classroom setting provides. Depending on the state, this was lost for over a year. A large learning gap resulted. Children were found to receive about one-third of what they ordinarily would have learned in a normal classroom school year.

A reprehensible consequence of pandemic online learning was that some socioeconomically disadvantaged children had no proper access to resources that assist with learning in reading and mathematics. In a March of 2022 source regarding the pandemic's impact on students, the Brookings Institution noted that the reading and math test scores plummeted for American students grades 3 through 8. One source noted that 4 in 10 American eighth graders failed to grasp basic math concepts. The state of Florida reopened most K-12 public and private schools in August of 2020. The state of New York fully reopened their schools in September of 2021. Various states presented data and reasons as to when it would be safe for the children and teachers to return to the physical classroom setting. This sometimes clashed with teachers' unions, specifically those who believed it to be unsafe to reopen site schools for the foreseeable future.

4

Clash of the Titans: Media Messaging

The term "media" is referred to as mass communications. Mass communications are carried out through the forms of newspapers, radio, television networks (telling a vision), vlogs, blogs, and other social media platforms (opinion and perception oriented). "Media" is derivative of the plural word, "medium", meaning intermediate or middle (of something or someone). How ironic that even in dark practices such as occultism, a medium (psychic or seer) is considered a person known to communicate with the spirit world on behalf of seekers (the tuned in audience). Those who come to these mediums are often desperate, thus they pay money, or render some other valued item (in this reference, "the mind") for the spiritual contact, and receive their sought information or confirmation (report). Furnishing one's mind sacrifices their thoughts for the medium's thoughts. The new thoughts and beliefs change attitudes and overall behaviors of the seekers. Many captivated participants become entranced with medium sources (information lines). The audience (customers), now hooked, continue coming back for additional downloads.

"Never let a crisis go to waste." This is an all-familiar phrase when reviewing the way important information is delivered to the public. Since inception, the job of a journalist or reporter was to provide current events and noteworthy information. One would agree that to maintain, stay relevant, and flourish in a media position, the individual must be presentable, knowledgeable, and able to captivate an audience's attention. These attributes keep the listener, reader, or viewer abreast of what they perceive they need to know, to do with that information what they need to do with it.

The art of the "wield" is a guileful maneuver. Wielders can craft messages to fit whatever they want their audience to hear, perceive, adopt beliefs on, and react to, in the manner of their liking. In desiring traction, masterful wielders use their tools to get it done through hot button, emotional topics, invoking outrage, anxiety, or fear. The outcome will be yet something else for wielders to report or comment on to their audience. There are reporters or commentators who do stick to the script. There are others who push the limits and expand, elevating opinions as factual. What is being added or taken away? Listening to the message and the manner of delivery, is often a revealer. There is nothing wrong with delivering facts using "personality"; however, facts should not be altered. The public must be discerning of speakers (mediums) who manipulate facts to fit particular audiences, and to receive negative emotional responses from those audiences for ratings' sake. In a turbulent time where Americans were searching for answers, the chance to pounce and capture minds at their most vulnerable, was at its peak. Several major news reporters, popular content creators on TikTok, YouTube, Twitter, and others, seized the moment, acquiring large financial gains. Conversely, many of their viewers and listeners were financially beset, or altogether drowning.

The Pew Research Center relayed that cable news networks revived in viewership as their ratings soared with the coverage of COVID-19. Once the viewers or listeners were tuned in, the networks had to keep their attention. Sources estimated that revenue for the three major cable news channels increased modestly in 2020 showing Fox News ($2.9 billion), CNN ($1.7 billion), and MSNBC ($1.1 billion). A valid concern was if platforms were providing facts to the best of the research found, as of the time reported on. Another voiced issue was that various platforms promoted open bias surrounding the virus. This included coaching the public on what they should believe and choices they should make, specifically once vaccines were available. Frequent disagreements and open rebuttals were observed, whether it was on the radio, television, or social media platforms. The regular presentations seen and heard on these outlets were evident of facts dipped in opinion and lies. An upcoming 2020 election seemed to add fuel to the flaming fire. It became judgmental to state where a virus allegedly originated and spread from. Facts later prevailed proving the initial alleged location of origin to be correct, and that there was actual merit for speculated cover-up concerns.

Critical thinkers wondered what media trance their fellow citizens were slipping into. It was as if some individuals and groups fell under a literal spell. Everything heard across the airwaves from someone of prominence or notoriety about the novel virus was taken as gospel truth because of "who" it came from. The push for groupthink and the visible evasion of those deemed to be stating or promoting misinformation or disinformation, pushed an influx of individuals to alternative social media platforms. The influential and social elite had to be (or publicly pretended to be) "on board" with every official protocol in place. If not, it would have been perceived by alleged handlers as them wanting people to pass away. How strange and limited in thinking to have such an extreme assumption. Having celebrity, or other high social status, does not necessitate a public statement or comment from these individuals on every single negative occurrence to express their disdain of said events.

It became common seeing marketed social media platforms display celebrities, thought leaders, activists, and the like, openly using their social influence to create friction, ridiculing those who were skeptical of vaccine efficacy, safety, and of certain mandates. Popular talk show hosts swayed their following audience in presumed efforts to "follow the science". If individuals were believed to not follow the science (in the specific area of the COVID-19 virus), those who knew them were urged to disassociate themselves and categorize those individuals as "COVID deniers". A witnessed odd and frequent occurrence was that certain comedian entertainers displayed discernible motives, or possible incentives, in convincing their audience to do and believe various COVID proclamations. This would appear to be outside of their purview. Famous music artists also became scientists and scholars overnight, wielding their influence to promote novel vaccines to their fans through lewd songs.

The elephant in the room was, pre-COVID, where was all of the advice and promotion of well documented health information that studies prove lead to lives saved by making healthier individuals for families and communities? To these entertainers, COVID suddenly became the only illness of focus that took valuable lives. Per data from the CDC, heart disease and cancer are still the leading causes of American deaths per year. Speculations swarmed of possible paid endorsements. This was due to the absurdity of entertainers promoting COVID inoculations when there were little to no reports of them recommending other vaccines in the past. It was transparent that America entered a "Club Shots Only" era. The shun button was pressed. Inoculation became the barrier to entry.

A common phrase among the spiritual is that, "There is power in the tongue". Repetition can lure droves. If someone of influence can utilize media to proclaim, write, type, like, react, and share things repeatedly, soon those topics will be discussed at family gatherings, worksites, and among inner circles as facts, without ever being proven. Emotional manipulation is targeted to those who may have experienced or be experiencing a void or form of trauma in their lives. COVID-19 caused, and manifested, traumatic experiences for many. The gravitation of these emotionally manipulated individuals and groups around the campfire of false, virally shared opinions, created a web of issues that caused implosion or explosion.

The CDC's website currently displays a section specifying how to address COVID-19 vaccine misinformation. They proclaim that "misinformation" arises when there are information gaps or unsettled science. They report that, as humans, we may share false information (misinformation) without intent to harm. They define "disinformation" as false information purposely created and disseminated with malicious intent. Joining along, the FDA also provided information on how to prevent the reported spread of rumors, misinformation and disinformation of science, medicine, and the FDA by utilizing Facebook, YouTube, Twitter, LinkedIn, and Instagram to report something as "inappropriate" content.

One thing of a surety, is that things carried out in the dark, can eventually come to the light. Hypocrisies regarding time frames of masking, social distancing, public gatherings, and vaccinations revealed a "rules for thee, not for me" mentality in elite circles. Throughout 2020 and 2021, several prominent political leaders, vocal on the importance of following the science and upholding pandemic restrictions, were discovered breaking those rules, traveling for leisure, and having personal parties and gatherings. One of those publicized parties was on Martha's Vineyard. This large gathering was reported as socially acceptable, presumedly because of the affluent guest list and hosts. An obvious message was conveyed. There was no negative media attention or rebuttals on COVID safety for those in the upper echelon. Somehow, other COVID restriction violators were reported on with vehement disgust. It was a repeated theme where normal citizens (who may have broken pandemic restrictions to gather for their planned events) were heavily scrutinized across the media, being vilified as super spreaders and COVID deniers. The over highlighting and media demonizing of the average citizen versus the leaders who promoted these restrictions, was hypocritically telling.

By two years into the pandemic, it was clear that several officials interviewed on major platforms, displayed inconsistencies. They had not openly apologized to the public for the mixed messaging on the virus. Does science change with time, particularly with a novel virus? Yes. Were there large swaths of COVID deniers or those that did not believe the illness existed? Time revealed that did not seem to be the case. Initially, there were groups that brushed off extra precautions, for whatever their reasons. Eventually, most people, even the initially skeptical, became convinced that the virus existed. Any able minded possible denier realized that there was something going on, whether they contracted the illness themselves, or had relatives, neighbors, friends, colleagues, church/mosque/temple members who fell ill, were hospitalized, or sadly passed away. Anyone and everyone was impacted.

The media is a powerful tool with the ability to impact and influence multitudes. Those who use it must exercise caution and wisdom. Using verbiage, body language, and insinuations with an audience to unneces-sarily invoke a negative, emotional response, is distasteful and beneath the standard of healthy journalism. On numerous occasions, viewers and listeners disclosed interpretations of beratement and misjudgment from the media. Many of these outlets professed inclusivity to all. The inclusivity was extended to the like-minded only. The hubris mentality of "just do what we say now", was the hailed motto. The "hustle" to drive higher ratings, grow income streams, popularity, and endorsements, should not have led reporters and commentators to shape content fueled with condescension of their neighboring American. These presentations further induced the strife, bitterness, prejudice, discrimination, and other hatefulness that many of them claim to be against.

It is imperative for the general public to gauge, not just what is being stated, but the manner in which it is being divulged. Always question the presenter's demeanor and disposition. Take note if the reporter or commentator attempts to persuade their audience into believing vulgar things about a person or subject, without acknowledging their audience's intellectual ability to conclude on the matter themselves. Be aware of presenters that covertly insult and condemn their audience for researching certain topics. Consuming information from media outlets must always accompany an individual's unbiased research of the presented subject matter.

5

Economic Repercussions

The United States economy experienced an intense shockwave. To provide financial assistance during the COVID-19 pandemic, former President Trump signed the Coronavirus Aid, Relief, and Economic Security (CARES) Act into law on March 27, 2020. The Senate approved the CARES Act in a unanimous vote, with 96 in favor. It was composed of $2.2 trillion in funding. The largest percentages of the funds went to assist small business owners ($377 billion) and direct payments to families ($293 billion). This aid assisted households, businesses, schools, unemployment, and more. On December 27, 2020, former President Trump signed the $910 billion Consolidated Appropriations Act (CAA) as another measure of ensuring that the American people would receive some form of immediate relief in such a trying time. A reported benefit to the CAA was that it provided an extra $300 a week in unemployment benefits for eleven weeks. The federal eviction moratorium was extended through January 31, 2021. Also, federal student loan payments were paused. The final aid was the American Rescue Plan Act (ARPA). This $1.9 trillion act was signed by President Biden on March 11, 2021. ARPA issued the highest amounts, in comparison to the previous acts, towards the areas of community development, vaccine development and distribution, schools, direct payments to families, and the United States Postal Service.

The weight of the COVID shutdowns resulted in various levels of devastation. Officials knew that something had to be done as soon as possible. This bipartisan belief was accurate as to the assumptions of what would happen to the American economy with continued shutdowns and limited financial flow. The attempt was to avoid the continued chaos of business closures, employees being furloughed or laid off, and citizens losing their homes from the inability to pay rent or mortgage. Interviews of various Americans in 2020 and early 2021 showed most in favor and appreciative of the funds received. Some business owners who received enough aid to remain in operation, were saved from closure. Other businesses and companies closed and never reopened, leading to mass waves of unemployment.

According to a September of 2022 report from the U.S. Census Bureau's 2021 Survey of Income and Program Participation, among those employed in January of 2020, adults 62 to 65 years old reported the most changes, with 4.6 percent stating they had retired early or planned to retire early, and 2.9 percent saying they had delayed or planned to delay their retirement. Record high numbers of workers with education jobs retired as a result of the pandemic. Per the U.S. Bureau of Labor Statistics, numerous businesses saw their supply chains disrupted, a declined demand for their products and services, shortages in supplies, and government mandated closures. Government mandated closures affected 48 percent of establishments in arts, recreation, and entertainment (the highest closure industry). The second highest closures were accommodation and food service establishments that employed over 5 million workers. Cities and states that would normally receive tourism, such as New York City, suffered loss of revenue. In April of 2021, the Office of the New York State Comptroller stated that tourism fell by 67 percent, having only 22.3 million visitors in 2020. This was a noticeable decrease from their 66.6 million visitors in 2019. California's tourism-related spending was reduced more than 50 percent in 2020, receiving around $65 billion in comparison to $144 billion in 2019. California tourism leaders beckoned for tourists to visit the state upon the June of 2021 official reopening of their restaurants, bars, museums, and other recreation sites.

By January of 2023, huge companies such as Meta, Google, Microsoft, and Amazon, eliminated thousands of jobs as a result of economic uncertainty and budget cuts. According to the May of 2023 employment report from the U.S. Department of Labor's Bureau of Labor Statistics, the unemployment rate rose by 0.3 percentage point to 3.7 percent. The issue of financial uncertainty continued to loom for some and resurrected for others. The year of 2022 welcomed higher prices for goods and services. Inflation was in full swing, tightening the grip on the American consumer and producer. "Inflation" was defined as an increase in the prices of goods and services over time due to an imbalance between demand and supply. The demand typically outpaces the rate of supply, which triggers the inflation. A December of 2022 report from the Roosevelt Institute, informed inflation to largely be attributed to supply chain issues. Other sources claimed that the relief funds poured into the economy, increased the demand for goods and services, which in turn, led to inflation. An additional believed cause was the cost and inadvertent repercussions of the Ukraine war. Since the war began, more than $75 billion in United States aid was provided.

In order to rein in inflation, the U. S. Federal Reserve decided that they needed to raise interest rates beginning March of 2022. Steady rate hikes followed. The negative impact of these raised rates was evident in the everyday cost of living that required frequent purchases. As the months passed, the purchase power of the American dollar continued to diminish. This was manifested in the prices of simple grocery items such as bread, eggs, milk, meat, and bottled water. American shoppers were quoted as having to go "store to store" to find products that were normally stocked at their first destination. Due to inflated prices, some shoppers verbalized making substitutions or altogether cut-outs of various items. According to a February 24, 2023 review from the Center for Strategic & International Studies, Russia and Ukraine accounted for one-third of global wheat trade, 75 percent of global sunflower oil trade, and 17 percent of the global maize trade. An observation of labels on various food items displayed substituted ingredients. Allegedly, this was a result of the shortages of former ingredients to make the products.

According to an April of 2023 CNBC Your Money Financial Confidence Survey, over 58 percent of Americans reported living paycheck to paycheck. The panic was that one-third of the participants had household incomes of six figures. About 61 percent of these six figure households believed inflation was a main contributor to their financial stress. A January of 2023 article from the National Public Radio (NPR) posited that more Americans were turning to credit cards to make up the difference, as interest rates and prices continued to climb. Around 46 percent carry a balance from month to month. In May of 2023, the Federal Reserve released data showing that the revolving debt increased by $17.6 billion in March of 2023. The United States revolving debt totaled $1.24 trillion.

Gasoline, by some reports, was at its highest in June of 2022, with an average price per gallon of just pennies under $5.00 per gallon. On March 8, 2022, USA Today informed that gas prices following the initiation of the war in Ukraine, were more expensive than during the 2008 recession. Furious drivers were seen on news interviews, and their own social media platforms, expressing their frustrations over whether they would have enough money for gasoline during their weekly commutes to and from work, their child's school, appointments, the grocery store, and other necessary places. Truck drivers were also feeling the squeeze.

An additional area of economic displeasure was centered around purchasing a home. A January 25, 2023 CNBC personal finance report relayed that about 92 percent of millennial homebuyers believed inflation had negatively impacted their purchase plans by causing increased housing prices. First- time home buyers composed just 26 percent of home purchases in 2022, a decrease from 34 percent in 2021. First- time home buyers were choosing to halt and allocate more time to saving for a larger down payment. January of 2023 brought some light at the end of the tunnel. The mortgage interest rate decreased from 7 percent in 2022. There was also not yet a housing market crash.

The U.S. Supreme Court ended the eviction moratoriums in August of 2021. Some states extended it. Current homeowners who were facing threats of eviction or foreclosure that did not willingly move out of their homes, were being foreclosed on due to non-payment. A common vocalized issue was that many home occupants were in houses they simply could not afford, possibly even pre-pandemic. Variable rate mortgages continued the trap of never getting caught up. In April of 2023, the major metropolitan cities with the highest foreclosures were New York City, Chicago, Los Angeles, and Houston.

According to the U.S. Department of Labor's Bureau of Labor Statistics (BLS), over 35 percent of households rent homes, per the 2017-2021 data. There persisted a myriad of concerns pertaining to the ability of renters getting their first, or a new apartment. Post-COVID, landlords were described as being more stringent during the tenant screening process. Income, job history, and previous evictions were heavily reviewed. Many landlords were also increasing rents to make up for the missed rental income unreceived during the pandemic. Renters who did not miss payments, disclosed that they still had to suffer for other tenants who did not or could not afford to pay their rent. Renters saw these escalated rent prices in 2022, even for one-bedroom apartments. By October of 2022, New York, New Jersey, and California were among the highest apartment priced states. A May of 2023 Zillow rental report noted a slight slowdown in rental price increases.

Sources continue to discredit that a recession is on the horizon. They proclaim that there was none during the pandemic; however, issues of economic uncertainty pressed on the backs of many American households, and the country itself. The U.S. national debt was estimated to be around $32 trillion dollars in May of 2023. Speculation of government shutdowns persisted. It was transparent that the nation's spending was out of control and needed honing in. A major issue of concern was that for years the nation's debt exceeded its gross domestic product (GDP). It looked as though the debt can was continually being kicked down the road. Servicing the high interest debt continued to be more costly per quarter as $213 billion in interest payments was paid on the national debt in the last quarter of 2022.

6

Where To from Here

Since the genesis of America's dismal encounter with COVID-19, conversations spread around the true purpose of the contrived COVID measures, mandates, and coerced compliance. Was this a "grand trial run" for something ahead far worse? Since October of 2021, vaccine mandates required by some employers, had cost tens of thousands of Americans their jobs. This included government and healthcare workers. The requirement was highly prevalent in states such as New York. In May of 2023, repeals were underway to no longer enforce vaccine mandates for employment in the state of New York; however, sources informed the employing facility could still implement their own policy requirements.

While incessantly reporting on the COVID-19 virus from March of 2020 through early 2022, there were other events transpiring, not as readily announced. The Stop Trading on Congressional Knowledge Act (STOCK Act) was passed by Congress and signed into law April 4, 2012 by former President Obama after years of allegations of insider trading from various Congress members. According to information from the Campaign Legal Center, Congress members continued complete stock transactions of over $150 million dollars. The members bought stocks in companies that they knew would increase in value during the pandemic.

These stocks included car manufacturers, healthcare companies, and remote work technologies. The average wage taxpayer was not privy to this information, thus, they did not experience the gains they possibly could have, if known. A September 13, 2022 New York Times article presented that over 90 current members of Congress bought or sold stock, bonds, or other financial assets, possibly in conflict of interest with their congressional work.

During and since the pandemic, strange food factory fires were reported with various food plants suffering losses. In June of 2023, lab-grown meat was approved for sale in the United States. The U.S. Department of Agriculture (USDA) reported that since 1961, the total meat consumption increased by 40 percent in America. In 2017, they cited that Americans were eating more meat than is recommended by national dietary guidelines. In 2020, chicken consumption elevated greatly. There were well-known fast-food restaurants vying for the public's business. Social media chicken sandwich challenges became popular, with individuals comparing the differences between the sandwich makers. Sources claimed that increased meat consumption and a growing population, was the reason behind an alternative and animal friendly method of meat production. Mass changes were in the works. The new normal had arrived. COVID-19 completely changed industries, relationships, finances, outlooks, and belief systems.

The World Health Organization (WHO) launched a new initiative for the improving of pandemic preparedness. This new initiative was called Preparedness and Resilience for Emerging Threats (PRET). PRET incorporates technical guidance and the latest tools and approaches for shared learning and collective action. The CDC established that they must be prepared to lead initiatives focusing on sharing scientific findings and data faster, enhancing laboratory science, developing a prepared workforce, and promoting results-based partnerships. The Response Ready Enterprise Data Integration platform (RREDI), considered to be the next generation of HHS Protect, is a secure decision-making and operations platform developed for the whole-of-government response to the COVID-19 pandemic. RREDI uses and integrates data from over 300 sources across federal, state, and local governments and the healthcare industry. It is accessible to 4,500 plus unique users across over 30 federal agencies, 56 states and territories, and the private sector.

A May 4, 2022 account from the Association of American Medical Colleges (AAMC) contended that confusion and hostility towards medical science did not solely begin with COVID. The report continued that science leaders in academia, and government, are recognizing that they must rise to the challenge of regaining credibility from the general public. This entails understanding several conditions, to include the forces and factors behind the public's distrust. The main force was a media environment that rewarded outrage, and the factor of the public being overwhelmed with too much information at a time. Dr. Janet Woodcock, deputy commissioner of the FDA, commented that, "The whole strength of science is that people who have different ideological bents can do experiments, transcend prior beliefs, and try to build a foundation of facts.".

The general trust of the American people to solve problems with non-biased solutions, must be at the forefront. To assume and spread falsities that someone or groups of people are less American by not agreeing with the esteemed choice of solutions, is preposterous. Often, problem solving can have various approaches and yield the same solutions. A solution-based mindset comes with hearing and respecting individuals whose method of solving the problem may differ from others. Finding common ground, without berating or shaming others, will garner the proper response from most citizens. Utilizing united front approaches with the goal of the public's health, livelihood, and well-being, are pertinent to a stable and thriving society.

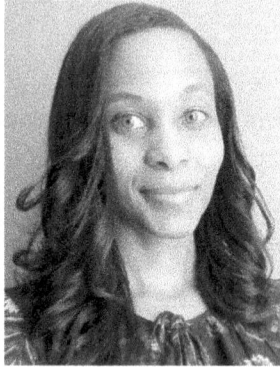

About the Author

C.F. Nero is an Alabama native. Since 2015, she has served numerous families as a licensed social worker in various capacities within her agency. She attended and graduated from Columbia Southern University with a Master of Public Administration in 2016 and the University of South Alabama with a Bachelor of Social Work in 2013. Her pillars are faith and family. She enjoys spending quality time with her husband and son.

Also by C.F. Nero

Is the concept of being a lady lost in modern culture? Is it possible to meet a woman who has not been swayed by mainstream trends and extreme antithetical belief systems? These are questions posed in conversation surrounding the present state of womanhood. It is critical to recognize the women who demonstrate upstanding character rather than fleeting trends. This book encourages evaluation of the messages delivered to women. The reader will be able to determine if popular messages are helping or harming the overall female image. Topics addressed include historical and scriptural references, marriage, destructive cultures, manipulative media messaging, and the feminist movement. This analysis ultimately explores the uniqueness of womanhood, and the ill willed, preconceived notions against women's distinction and significance.

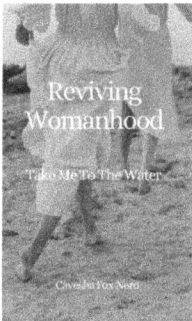

Reviving Womanhood

This book is for young, middle, and senior aged ladies who desire to learn and grow in their God created purpose. It is for females searching for or embracing the peculiar feminine qualities and functions that make women as special as they are.

www.ingramcontent.com/pod-product-compliance
Lightning Source LLC
Chambersburg PA
CBHW060531280326
41933CB00014B/3132